The Two Week Transformation

Your kick-start to a healthier lifestyle!

by Dan DeFigio

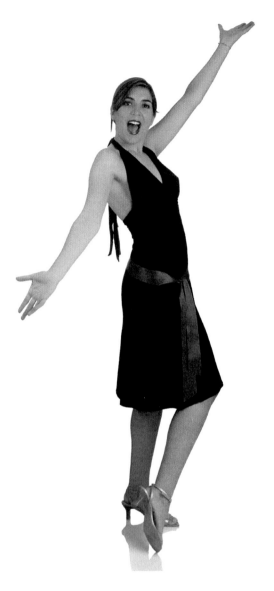

TwoWeekTransformation.com

The Two Week Transformation is a simple, straightforward system that will start to change your body in just two weeks – you'll lose a pants size in two weeks, guaranteed!

So many times people beg me to "Just tell me what to do and I'll do it!"

So here you go:
A short, easy booklet that explains exactly what to do for two disciplined weeks.

If you follow this two-week plan exactly, I guarantee that you will lose at least one pants size, and you will feel fantastic!

This simple guide tells you exactly what to do for the next two weeks -- what you should (and shouldn't) eat, recommended supplements, exercise tips, and some extra credit options too, if you want to really get serious.
You can do ANYTHING for two weeks, can't you? Get the kick start you need, and start your Two Week Transformation right now!

Disclaimer and Terms of Use

The author and the publisher do not hold any responsibility for errors, omissions, or interpretation of the subject matter herein, and specifically disclaim any responsibility for the safety or appropriateness of any dietary advice or exercise advice presented in this book. This book is presented for informational purposes only. Always consult a qualified health care practitioner before beginning any diet or exercise program.

Table of Contents

Introduction

Are you ready for the NEW YOU?
The Two Week Transformation is a simple, proven system that will change your body in just two weeks!

What it is

So many times people beg me to "Just tell me what to do and I'll do it!"

So here you go:
A few sheets of paper that explain exactly what to do (and what NOT to do) for two disciplined weeks. Whether you call it a detox, a kickstart, a diet plan, or a lifestyle improvement program, ***The Two Week Transformation*** is here to help you get started down the right path to weight loss, energy, and better health!

If you follow this two-week plan exactly, I guarantee that you will lose at least one pants size, and you will feel fantastic!

What it's not

The Two Week Transformation is not a secret "miracle diet" that was developed by time-traveling scientists from another planet who are just now making it available to a select few for five easy payments of $19.95. It is not an infomercial WünderGizmo that promises to unleash massive physiological reactions never before witnessed in nature. It is not a diet book with hundreds of confusing pages that conflict with the last miracle diet you tried. There are no miserable "phases" to go through, no food-weighing, no calorie-tracking, and no carb-counting. You will not find perplexing scientific gobbledygook that means nothing to you – Just a detailed, specific system of what to do to lose (at least) a pants size in two weeks. And you'll feel great while you do it!

What are you waiting for?

I will encourage you to read through this book and get started on your Transformation right away. Don't tell yourself, "I'll start on Monday," or that you're going to "wait until things calm down at work." You'll never get started that way! Write this down and put it where you can see it several times per day:

Being healthy or being unhealthy is a series of ongoing decisions over your entire lifetime. You are a product of what you do most of the time. Make every decision count, because it does.

If you don't make healthy decisions because you're waiting for a time in your life when you never have anything going on,

2

there's nothing stressful happening, and you magically have more time to focus on yourself instead of caring for other people, you will be waiting forever. That fairy tale isn't happening. Ever. The "perfect time" to start acting differently is RIGHT NOW, because it's the only time you'll ever have!

The best advice in the world is useless until it is implemented. If reading diet books made people thin and healthy, Americans would be the thinnest people in the history of the world. You do not improve your body because you read a self-help book or went to see a motivational speaker. You will only achieve positive, permanent change when you
START DOING THINGS DIFFERENTLY.

So start being different RIGHT NOW – Ready, set, go!

BONUS

Simple exercise is an important part of health, wellness, and weight loss. Before you continue reading, please visit
TwoWeekTransformation.com to gain free access to proper exercise instruction – and several additional bonuses – just because I want to help you succeed in every way I can.

What you may or may not know

There is a lot of conflicting information concerning health and weight loss, and people often get confused about what they should or should not be doing, so they end up doing nothing. In order to shed some light on some basic nutrition principles, here are a few things you should know for long-term nutrition success:

Meal timing

Most people have heard that you should eat five or six small meals each day. If you go more than three or four hours without eating, your body begins holding on to its fat stores as a protection against starvation. In order to get your body to willingly give up its stored fat, you need to eat a small amount of food every three or four hours.

When I first started helping people with nutrition in 1993, I figured that getting folks to eat the right things would be the biggest challenge, but I was wrong -- it's **timing** that gives people trouble. People tend to stay so busy all day that one of the last things that they think about is feeding themselves. When you do not eat often enough during the day, by the time you get home from work, your brain realizes that you have not eaten enough calories yet, and turns on the ravenous appetite. Then you eat whatever you can get your hands on quickly, and way too much of it. Eating often enough can keep you from making frantic, foolish choices.

Eating frequently will help to keep your blood sugar levels more even throughout day. If you go too long without eating, your blood sugar levels fall too low and you'll crash – complete with low energy, difficulty concentrating, irritability, etc. When you eat too much at one time, or when you eat processed carbohydrates without protein or fat, you'll get a rapid rise in blood sugar levels. This forces your body to release too much insulin, which:

1. Promotes fat storage
2. Contributes to insulin resistance and Type 2 Diabetes
3. Makes you sleepy later on
4. Prevents fat burning

You can read more about carbohydrates and insulin control in **Beating Sugar Addiction For Dummies** (BeatingSugarAddiction.com).

Protein

Proteins are the building blocks for many parts of our bodies. Muscles, hemoglobin, enzymes, genes, and immune system cells are all made from proteins. If you don't eat enough protein, you compromise your body's production of these vital structures.

You should try to eat a protein source every time you eat. This will help stabilize your blood sugar and insulin, keep you satisfied for a longer period of time, and ensure that you're getting enough dietary protein for maximum health and vitality.

Here are some good protein sources:

- Powdered whey protein (you'll find many uses for whey protein in my **Beyond Smoothies** book at BeyondSmoothies.us)
- Egg
- Fish
- Lean meats
- Skinless poultry
- Skim dairy
- Soy
- Legumes and nuts

Three or four ounces (the size of your palm or a deck of cards) of fish, meat, or poultry typically has 20-25 grams of protein. Legumes and nuts vary in their protein content, so read your labels.

Water

Water should be the mainstay of your beverages throughout the day. Being dehydrated leads to low energy, decreased mental function, and food cravings. Drink at least 64 ounces of distilled water every day. If you love the fizz of soda, drink mineral water instead. You can flavor it with citrus if you like.

Whole Foods

Do your best to eat foods in their natural state, with as little processing and possible. Processed foods are loaded with artificial ingredients, modified fats, sugars, preservatives, and lots of chemicals that do not lead to good health.

Whole foods are found in nature, they haven't been processed, the nutrients remain intact, and they don't contain unhealthy chemicals.

Which has more nutrients – a package of peanut butter crackers, or an apple topped with organic peanut butter? Which has more chemicals? If it comes in a wrapper, try to find a healthier alternative.

THE PLAN

Here's the plan to lose a pants size in two weeks, laid out in two simple "Don't Do This" and "Do This" sections.

The DON'T List

What you promise NOT to eat for the next two weeks:

1. No flour products – bread, pasta, bakery stuff, etc. No processed carbs – only vegetables and fruits for two weeks.

> Processed carbohydrates are low in nutrients and fiber and high in calories. They also cause a rapid rise in blood sugar levels, eliciting a large insulin response. This promotes fat storage, makes you sleepy, increases food cravings, and over time can cause insulin resistance and diabetes.

2. Only drink water, tea, or coffee. No fruit juice, alcohol, sodas, sugar-laden frappuccinos, or diet drinks (see below) for two weeks. If you must sweeten your water or tea, use a slice or two of fresh citrus or a sprinkle of stevia powder.

> Drinking calories is a sure way to pack on the pounds. Sugar-laden fruit juice or sweetened drinks supply lots of calories and sugar, making weight loss difficult if not

impossible. Fructose overload (from too much fruit juice or high-fructose corn syrup) causes fat storage and increased appetite.

3. No food after 7:00 pm. Period. If you get home late from work at 7:01, you missed the dinner bus. You should have planned ahead.

Eat to fuel what you're going to do for the next 3 or 4 hours. If your after-dinner plans are sitting on the couch and watching a movie before going to bed, you don't need many calories. Under-eating during the day leads to over-eating at night and triggers cravings for sugar. Late-night eating leads to all those unused calories being stored as fat.

4. No sugar, no corn syrup.

Sugar overload is a driving force behind obesity, diabetes, liver disease, autoimmune disorders, chronic fatigue, hypothyroid disease, high cholesterol, osteoporosis, and metabolic syndrome. It acts on the same pleasure center of the brain as alcohol and heroin, so the more you eat, the more you want. The less sugar you eat, the better!

Some other words manufacturers use for sugars are:

Glycerine or Glycerol
Dextrin, Dextrose, or Polydextrose
Cane juice

Corn sweeteners
Molasses
Beet sugar
Fructose
Barley malt
Sorbitol
Fruit juice concentrate
Turbinado
Xylitol

If you're a Choco-holic or a sugar addict, check out **BeatingSugarAddiction.com** for lots of tips for successfully getting off sugar.

5. Stay away from artificial sweeteners like aspartame (Nutrasweet), MSG, sucralose (Splenda), and saccharin (Sweet n' Low).

Chemical sweeteners increase appetite and can cause brain damage (see **GettingFit.com/sweeteners**).

6. No trans-fats (hydrogenated oils). This means no fried food, no fake peanut butter, no margarine, no Crisco.

I think by now most people know that trans fats wreak havoc on your cardiovascular health. Trans fats (a.k.a. *hydrogenated fats*) are created when fats are over-heated (such as deep-frying). They can also be artificially added to foods in order to delay spoilage. Trans fats raise LDL (bad) cholesterol, lower LDL (good) cholesterol, and increase triglycerides – all bad news for your arteries!

1. **Eat breakfast within 30 minutes of getting up in the morning.**

> Yes, you have to. If you absolutely hate eating food in the morning, make a green drink instead (see "Extra Credit" below). Breakfast – especially a high-protein breakfast – raises your metabolism and increases your calorie burn for the whole day! It will also increase your energy and improve your mental performance.

2. **Take the right multi-vitamin/mineral supplement with breakfast every day.**

> Ensuring you have enough essential nutrients will maximize your health and minimize your food cravings. For best results, add 2 grams of fish oil capsules daily (if you use blood-thinning medication, consult a qualified professional first). It's important to get the right kind -- Recommended brands (at a discount!) are available at **GettingFit.com/shop**.

3. **Move in the morning!**

> Take a walk for a few minutes before breakfast. Or get up and stretch. If you're a cardio person, get on the elliptical, or go for a quick jog. Spend 5 minutes doing deep breathing practice before you get out of bed. Or just get up and march in place for 2 minutes. Do something! Activity early in the

day will energize you and increase your metabolism.

Don't forget to get your free exercise programs from TwoWeekTransformation.com!

4. **Protein should come from "clean" animals:**

- Pasture-fed chicken and eggs, raised without hormones or antibiotics.
- Beef should be grass-fed and hormone-free.
- Choose wild-caught fish instead of farmed.
- Organic, non-GMO soy and nuts if you're a vegetarian.
- Powdered whey protein is also an option – hormone-free, and without additives or artificial sweeteners, of course.

5. **Vegetables and fruits should be organic, and local whenever possible.**

Organic produce is natural (non-genetically modified) and grown without pesticides and chemical fertilizers. Buy local food when you can – it's fresher, it will have more nutrients, and you'll support local farms. Do you really need to buy a red pepper shipped from Holland?

6. **Plan your food in advance.**

   Whether you do it the night before, or on Sunday for the whole upcoming week, you need to know what you're going to eat before it's time to eat!

More Advice

Don't sabotage yourself! Don't keep junk food in the house or at work. If a food (or beverage) isn't nutritious and isn't helping you reach your goal, why the hell do you have it?

- *"I hate wasting food."*
  Me too. Give it away!

- *"My kid / husband / roommate likes these."*
  Grownups can get their own junk food if they really want it. It's not your job to enable their poor nutrition. Don't feed your kids junk food whether they want it or not. You're responsible for their health!

- *"It's for special occasions, like when I have a bad day at work."*
  Giving yourself a treat once in awhile is fine. When you decide it's treat time, go buy one - don't keep any handy in the house. DO NOT use junk food to medicate yourself after a stressful day!

Food decisions in the kitchen need to be foolproof. When you get home late from work and are starving, don't make yourself decide between ice cream and spinach. Keep junk food out of the house so you're not tempted, and keep healthy, ready-to-eat foods on hand for times when you don't have time to cook.

Keep cooked grains, like brown rice or quinoa, in the refrigerator. Your meal is already halfway done!

Keep bags of frozen organic vegetables stocked in the freezer for days when you don't have fresh produce. These frozen veggies are great for a quick snack or stir fry.

Don't try to make things too complicated, or worry too much about insignificant details. Keep things simple so you can be consistent!

Extra credit

Start each day with a nutrient-packed green drink. You can juice your own vegetables and fruits, or you can use Univera's Metagreens powder: **GettingFit.com/shop**

Add a probiotic supplement to your multi-vitamin and fish oil regimen: **GettingFit.com/probiotics**

Lots of people get a low-grade allergic response to dairy. So if you're feeling particularly brave or motivated, try going dairy-free for two weeks and see how you feel.

Concerning exercise: The best way to lose weight and really get in shape is to do short bouts of high-intensity exercise. Work short, but work hard. But remember that any exercise is better than none, so if higher-intensity exercise is not appropriate for you, try lower-intensity activities (like walking or swimming) for longer periods of time.

Don't forget to get all your free bonus material, including fat-blasting exercise programs, at TwoWeekTransformation.com!

Did you enjoy this book?

Please leave a review on Amazon – let everyone know what you liked about

The Two Week Transformation!

 Amazon.com/gp/css/order-history
Then click on "*Digital Orders*"

SPREAD THE WORD:

**Word-of-mouth is vital to independent authors!
Please post a link to
TwoWeekTransformation.com on your
Facebook and Twitter pages!**

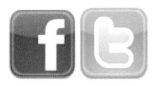

About the author

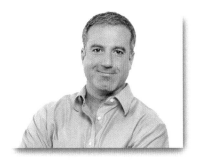 Dan DeFigio is a recognized exercise and nutrition expert who has been featured on *The Dr. Phil Show*, in *SELF magazine* and *MD News*, on the cover of *Personal Trainer Magazine*, and a number of other publications, television shows, and radio broadcasts.

Since 1993, Dan DeFigio has been on the cutting edge of exercise and nutrition science, leading celebrities, health professionals, and couch potatoes alike down the road to success. His expertise has been shared with thousands of clients and millions of readers worldwide. Dan's most popular book is **Beating Sugar Addiction For Dummies**, at BeatingSugarAddiction.com.

In addition to teaching exercise and nutrition, Dan is a former competitive mixed-martial-arts fighter, culminating his career with a win at the 2000 Pan American Games. Some also say he is quite a piano player.